Welcome

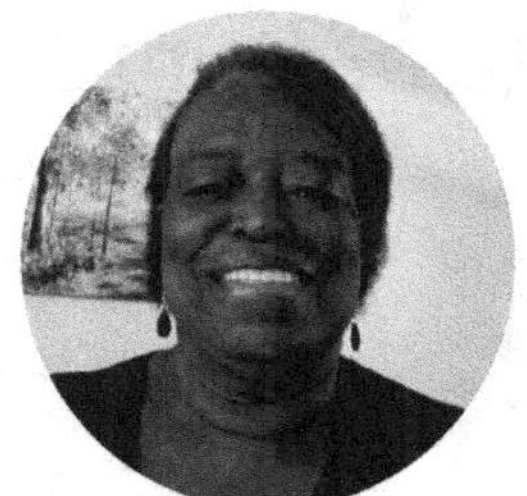

Hello, I am

Desiree Rose

I am your Author, and I have been Publishing books on the KDP Platform for two years. I am a Retired Nurse, and I have had the pleasure to serve over fifty years in the medical field. I have also been able to share my knowledge by training the next generation of nurses. I am a mother of two children, and two grandchildren, with a great granddaughter on the way. I am also in my seventies, managing my diabetes with the help of my medical team. I am no expert, but I hope that this book will encourage you in some small way.

Table of Contents

A Healthy Guide for Seniors

Living with Diabetes
Chapter: 1 *Understanding Diabetes*

Diabetes is a chronic medical condition that affects how your body processes glucose, the primary source of energy for your cells. In a healthy individual, the hormone insulin, produced by the pancreas, helps move glucose from the bloodstream into the cells. However, in people with diabetes, this process is impaired. There are two main types of diabetes: Type 1, which is often diagnosed in childhood and involves the body not producing insulin, and Type 2, which is more common in seniors and is characterized by insulin resistance or inadequate insulin production. Understanding these differences is crucial for managing the disease effectively.

Type 2 diabetes is particularly prevalent among seniors and is often associated with factors like obesity, physical inactivity, and genetic predisposition. As people age, their bodies may become less efficient at using insulin, leading to elevated blood sugar levels. It is important for seniors to recognize the symptoms of diabetes, which can include increased thirst, frequent urination, unexplained weight loss, fatigue, and blurred vision. Regular monitoring of blood sugar levels can help in detecting diabetes early, allowing for timely intervention and management.

Managing diabetes involves a combination of lifestyle changes and, in some cases, medication. A balanced diet that focuses on whole foods, low in sugar and refined carbohydrates, can significantly improve blood sugar control. Seniors should aim to include plenty of vegetables, lean proteins, healthy fats, and whole grains in their meals. Additionally, regular physical activity is vital. Engaging in activities such as walking, swimming, or even gentle stretching can help lower blood sugar levels and improve overall health. It's also essential for seniors with diabetes to maintain regular check-ups with their healthcare providers. These visits can help monitor

complications associated with diabetes, such as heart disease, kidney damage, and neuropathy. Healthcare professionals can provide personalized advice on managing diabetes, including medication adjustments and lifestyle recommendations. Being proactive about health can empower seniors to take control of their diabetes and reduce the risk of complications.

Finally, emotional well-being plays a significant role in managing diabetes. The diagnosis can be overwhelming, and seniors may experience feelings of isolation or anxiety. Support groups, whether in-person or online, can provide valuable resources and a sense of community. Connecting with others who share similar experiences can foster resilience and encourage positive health behaviors. By prioritizing both physical and emotional health, seniors can lead fulfilling lives while managing their diabetes effectively.

Types of Diabetes

Diabetes is a chronic condition that affects how your body processes glucose, a type of sugar that serves as a primary energy source. There are several types of diabetes, each with its own causes, risk factors, and management strategies. Understanding the different types is crucial for seniors as it can help them make informed decisions about their health and lifestyle. The main types of diabetes include Type 1 diabetes, Type 2 diabetes, and gestational diabetes, along with a less common form known as latent autoimmune diabetes in adults (LADA).

Type 1 diabetes is an autoimmune condition where the body's immune system attacks insulin-producing cells in the pancreas. This results in little to no insulin production, making it necessary for individuals with Type 1 diabetes to rely on insulin injections or an insulin pump for management. While Type 1 diabetes typically develops in childhood or adolescence, it can occur in adults as well. Seniors diagnosed with Type 1 diabetes must be vigilant about monitoring their blood sugar levels, adhering to insulin therapy, and managing their diet to maintain stable glucose levels.

Type 2 diabetes is the most prevalent form of the disease, accounting for approximately 90% of all diabetes cases. It usually develops when the body becomes resistant to insulin or when the pancreas fails to produce enough insulin. This type of diabetes is often linked to lifestyle factors such as obesity, physical inactivity, and poor diet. Seniors are at a higher risk for Type 2 diabetes due to age-related changes in metabolism and muscle mass. Management typically includes lifestyle modifications such as dietary changes, regular physical activity, and, if necessary, medication to help regulate blood sugar levels.

Gestational diabetes occurs during pregnancy when the body is unable to produce enough insulin to meet the increased demands. While this type typically resolves after childbirth, it can increase the risk of developing Type 2 diabetes later in life. Although gestational diabetes primarily affects pregnant women, seniors who have experienced it in the past should be aware of their increased risk for future diabetes and take proactive steps to monitor their health. Regular check-ups and blood sugar screenings are essential for early detection and management.

Latent autoimmune diabetes in adults (LADA) is a form of diabetes that shares characteristics of both Type 1 and Type 2 diabetes. It is often misdiagnosed as Type 2 diabetes because it develops gradually and typically occurs in adults over 30. However, individuals with LADA are often insulin-dependent within a few years of diagnosis. For seniors, recognizing the symptoms and understanding the distinction between LADA and other types of diabetes is important for proper management. Early diagnosis and appropriate treatment can help prevent complications and lead to better health outcomes.

The Importance of Blood Sugar Management

Managing blood sugar levels is crucial for seniors living with diabetes, as it directly impacts overall health and well-being. High blood sugar, or hyperglycemia, can lead to a variety of complications, including heart disease, nerve damage, kidney issues, and vision problems. Conversely, low blood sugar, or hypoglycemia, can cause confusion, dizziness, and even loss of consciousness. Understanding how to maintain balanced blood sugar levels is essential for preventing these serious health concerns and ensuring a better quality of life.

One of the key aspects of blood sugar management is regular monitoring. Seniors should work with their healthcare providers to determine the most appropriate blood glucose targets and the frequency of testing. Monitoring not only helps in adjusting dietary choices but also aids in understanding how different foods, activities, and medications affect blood glucose levels. Keeping a detailed log can provide valuable insights into patterns, enabling seniors to make informed decisions about their lifestyle choices and treatment plans.

Diet plays a significant role in blood sugar management. Seniors should focus on a balanced diet that includes a variety of whole grains, lean proteins, healthy fats, and plenty of fruits and vegetables. Carbohydrate counting can be a useful strategy, as it helps in understanding how different carbohydrates impact blood sugar levels. Additionally, portion control is essential, as overeating can lead to spikes in blood glucose. Staying hydrated and limiting sugary beverages also contribute to better blood sugar control.

Physical activity is another important factor in managing blood sugar. Regular exercise can enhance insulin sensitivity, making it easier for the body to use glucose effectively. Seniors should aim for at least 150 minutes of moderate aerobic activity each week, alongside strength training exercises at least twice a week. Engaging in activities such as walking, swimming, or dancing not only helps regulate blood sugar but also promotes cardiovascular health, mobility, and mental well-being.

Finally, medication management is crucial for seniors with diabetes. Many may require insulin or oral medications to help control their blood sugar levels. It is important for seniors to understand their medications, including how they work and the potential side effects. Regular consultations with healthcare providers can ensure that medication regimens are adjusted as needed based on blood sugar readings and lifestyle changes. By taking a proactive approach to blood sugar management, seniors can significantly improve their health outcomes and enjoy a more active, fulfilling life.

Chapter 2: Nutrition and Meal Planning
Building a Balanced Plate

Building a balanced plate is essential for managing diabetes effectively, particularly for seniors who may have unique dietary needs and health considerations. A balanced plate incorporates a variety of food groups in appropriate proportions, which not only helps in blood sugar management but also ensures that seniors receive the nutrients necessary for overall well-being. Understanding how to portion meals can empower individuals to make healthier choices that align with their diabetes management goals.

To create a balanced plate, it is important to include a combination of carbohydrates, proteins, and healthy fats. Carbohydrates should come primarily from whole grains, fruits, and non-starchy vegetables, as these sources provide fiber that aids digestion and helps regulate blood sugar levels. Foods like brown rice, quinoa, and whole grain bread offer complex carbohydrates, which digest more slowly than simple carbohydrates, leading to a steadier release of glucose into the bloodstream. Seniors should aim to fill about one-quarter of their plate with these healthy carbohydrate sources.

Proteins play a crucial role in maintaining muscle mass, especially for seniors who may be at risk of muscle loss. Lean proteins, such as chicken, turkey, fish, beans, and legumes, are excellent choices that can be included in meals. Aiming to fill another quarter of the plate

with
protein not only helps in managing hunger but also supports overall health. Additionally, incorporating plant-based proteins can provide added benefits, such as lowering cholesterol levels and reducing the risk of heart disease, which is particularly important for those with diabetes.

Healthy fats are also a vital component of a balanced plate. These fats, found in foods like avocados, nuts, seeds, and olive oil, can help improve heart health and provide essential fatty acids that the body needs. Filling a small portion of the plate with healthy fats can enhance the flavor of meals while contributing to satiety. Seniors should be mindful of portion sizes, as fats are calorie-dense, but including these fats in moderation can support a nutritious diet without negatively impacting blood sugar levels.

Lastly, hydration and mindful eating are important aspects to consider when building a balanced plate. Seniors should not overlook the significance of water intake, as staying hydrated is essential for overall health, especially in managing diabetes. Additionally, practicing mindful eating—taking the time to savor each bite and listen to hunger cues— can help seniors better manage portion sizes and improve their relationship with food. By focusing on a balanced plate and incorporating these principles, diabetic seniors can create enjoyable and healthful meals that support their diabetes management and enhance their quality of life.

Carbohydrates and Their Impact

Carbohydrates are one of the three macronutrients essential for our body's functioning, alongside proteins and fats. For seniors managing diabetes, understanding how carbohydrates affect blood sugar levels is crucial. Carbohydrates are found in various foods, including grains, fruits, vegetables, and dairy products. They are the body's primary source of energy, but not all carbohydrates are created equal. Simple carbohydrates, found in sugary foods and refined grains, can cause rapid spikes in blood sugar levels, while complex carbohydrates, found in whole grains, legumes, and vegetables, are digested more slowly, leading to a steadier release of glucose into the bloodstream.

When it comes to diabetes management, the quality and quantity of carbohydrates are vital. Foods high in fiber, such as whole grains, fruits, and vegetables, are beneficial for maintaining stable blood sugar levels. Fiber slows digestion and the absorption of sugar, which can help prevent the sharp increases in blood glucose that can be harmful to diabetics. Additionally, incorporating low-glycemic index foods into the diet can be particularly advantageous. These foods have a slower, more gradual effect on blood sugar levels, making them a preferable choice for seniors with diabetes.

Portion control is another factor that diabetic seniors must consider when consuming carbohydrates. Understanding serving sizes and how they translate into carbohydrate intake can help manage blood glucose levels more effectively. Using tools such as measuring cups or carbohydrate counting apps can assist in making informed choices. It is also helpful to balance carbohydrate intake with protein and healthy fats, which can contribute to a more stable blood sugar response. This balance can enhance satiety and reduce the likelihood of overeating, which is particularly important for seniors who may have different energy needs.

Planning meals ahead of time can also play a significant role in managing carbohydrate intake. By preparing meals that include a variety of nutrient-dense foods, seniors can ensure they are consuming the right types and amounts of carbohydrates. This practice not only helps in regulating blood sugar levels but also promotes overall health. Meal prepping can involve cooking in batches, portioning out meals, and keeping healthy snacks on hand. Being proactive in meal planning can reduce the temptation to reach for quick, high-sugar options when hunger strikes.

Finally, staying informed about the latest nutritional guidelines and recommendations can empower seniors to make healthier choices regarding carbohydrates. Consulting with healthcare professionals, such as registered dietitians, can provide personalized advice tailored to individual health needs. Educational resources, workshops, and support groups can also offer valuable information and encouragement. By understanding the role of carbohydrates in their diet, diabetic seniors can take charge of their health and enjoy a better quality of life.

Reading Nutrition Labels

Reading nutrition labels is an essential skill for diabetic seniors, as it empowers individuals to make informed choices about their food intake. Nutrition labels provide crucial information about the contents of food products, helping to identify carbohydrates, sugars, and other nutritional components that can affect blood sugar levels. Understanding how to read these labels can lead to better management of diabetes and overall health.

One of the first steps in reading nutrition labels is to look at the serving size. Serving sizes are standardized measurements that indicate the amount of food that the nutritional information refers to. It is vital to compare the serving size on the label with the actual amount you plan to consume. For example, if a label lists a serving size as one cup but you consume two cups, you need to double the nutritional values, particularly carbohydrates and sugars, to understand their impact on your blood glucose.

Next, focus on the total carbohydrates section of the nutrition label. Carbohydrates are the primary nutrient that affects blood sugar levels, and understanding this figure is crucial for diabetes management. The total carbohydrates listed includes sugars, starches, and fiber. For diabetic seniors, it is particularly important to differentiate between total carbohydrates and added sugars. Added sugars can significantly raise blood sugar levels, so choosing foods with lower added sugars is essential for maintaining stable glucose levels.

Another important aspect to consider is dietary fiber. Foods high in fiber can help regulate blood sugar levels by slowing the absorption of sugar into the bloodstream. When reading labels, look for products that contain at least three grams of dietary fiber per serving. Foods rich in fiber, such as whole grains, fruits, and vegetables, not only support blood sugar control but also promote digestive health, which can be particularly beneficial for seniors.

Lastly, pay attention to other nutrients and ingredients listed on the label. Look for healthy fats, protein content, and sodium levels, as these factors can also impact overall health and diabetes management. Choosing foods with healthier fat sources, adequate protein, and lower sodium can lead to a more balanced diet. Additionally, familiarize yourself with any unfamiliar ingredients, as some may contain hidden sugars or unhealthy additives. By becoming proficient in reading nutrition labels, diabetic seniors can enhance their dietary choices, leading to improved health outcomes and a better quality of life.

Meal Timing and Frequency

Meal timing and frequency play a crucial role in managing diabetes, especially for seniors. As we age, our metabolism changes, and our bodies may respond differently to food intake. For individuals with diabetes, understanding how and when to eat can help maintain stable blood sugar levels, prevent spikes and crashes, and promote overall well-being. Establishing a routine that includes regular meals and snacks can be beneficial for blood sugar control and can contribute to a more balanced dietary approach.

Consistent meal timing helps regulate the body's internal clock and can enhance insulin sensitivity. For seniors, it is often recommended to eat at regular intervals throughout the day. This might include three balanced meals and one or two healthy snacks. By spacing meals evenly, seniors can help ensure that their blood sugar levels remain stable. This routine can also help prevent the temptation to overeat or indulge in unhealthy snacks due to prolonged periods of hunger.

Choosing the right foods is essential when considering meal frequency. Complex carbohydrates, lean proteins, and healthy fats should be the foundation of each meal. Seniors should focus on high-fiber foods such as whole grains, fruits, and vegetables, as these can help slow the absorption of sugar into the bloodstream. Incorporating protein in each meal can also promote satiety, making it less likely for individuals to experience cravings or excessive hunger between meals.

In addition to what is eaten, how meals are structured can also impact blood sugar levels. Eating smaller, more frequent meals can be beneficial for seniors with diabetes. This approach can help reduce the likelihood of large blood sugar spikes that may occur after consuming a large meal. For those who find it challenging to consume larger portions, smaller meals can also be easier to digest and more enjoyable, contributing to better nutrient absorption and overall health.

Lastly, it is important for seniors to listen to their bodies and adapt their meal timing and frequency as needed. Factors such as physical activity, medication schedules, and personal preferences can influence dietary choices. Keeping a food diary may help individuals track their eating patterns and understand how different foods affect their blood sugar levels. Consulting with healthcare providers or dietitians can provide personalized guidance, ensuring that each senior can create a meal plan that supports their unique health needs while managing diabetes effectively.

Chapter 3: Healthy Food Choices
Incorporating Whole Foods

Incorporating whole foods into the diets of diabetic seniors is a vital step toward managing blood sugar levels while promoting overall health. Whole foods, such as fruits, vegetables, whole grains, lean proteins, and healthy fats, provide essential nutrients without the added sugars and unhealthy fats often found in processed foods. By emphasizing these natural options, seniors can enhance their nutritional intake, improve their energy levels, and support their immune systems, all of which are crucial for maintaining health and vitality.

One of the primary benefits of whole foods is their high fiber content, which plays a significant role in blood sugar management. Foods like beans, lentils, oats, and vegetables are rich in fiber, helping to slow the absorption of glucose into the bloodstream. This gradual release helps to prevent spikes in blood sugar levels, making it easier for seniors to maintain stable readings throughout the day. Moreover, fiber aids in digestion, promoting regularity and reducing the risk of constipation, a common concern among the elderly.

In addition to fiber, whole foods are abundant in vitamins and minerals that support various bodily functions. For instance, leafy greens such as spinach and kale are packed with vitamins A, C, and K, as well as important minerals like calcium and iron. These nutrients are essential for maintaining strong bones, enhancing vision, and supporting heart health. Seniors who incorporate a variety of whole foods into their diets can benefit from a broader spectrum of nutrients that contribute to overall well-being and reduce the risk of chronic diseases.

Meal planning that focuses on whole foods can also be a straightforward way for diabetic seniors to control their portions and make healthier food choices. Preparing meals that include a balance of proteins, healthy fats, and complex carbohydrates can lead to satisfying and nutritious dishes. For example, a meal could consist of grilled chicken served with quinoa and a side of steamed vegetables. Such combinations not only provide essential nutrients but also help seniors feel full and satisfied, reducing the temptation to reach for unhealthy snacks.

Finally, making the shift to whole foods does not need to be overwhelming. Seniors can start by gradually replacing processed foods with whole food alternatives. This could involve simple changes, such as choosing brown rice instead of white rice or snacking on fresh fruits and nuts instead of sugary snacks. By taking small steps, seniors can develop a sustainable approach to

eating that enhances their health and quality of life. Embracing whole foods is a powerful strategy for managing diabetes and enjoying a vibrant, healthy lifestyle.

The Role of Fiber

Fiber plays a crucial role in the dietary management of diabetes, especially for seniors. It is a type of carbohydrate that the body cannot digest, which means it does not raise blood sugar levels the way other carbohydrates do. For seniors, incorporating fiber into their diets can help regulate blood glucose levels, improve digestive health, and provide a sense of fullness that can aid in weight management. This is particularly important for older adults who may be at risk for obesity or metabolic syndrome, conditions that can complicate diabetes management.

There are two main types of dietary fiber: soluble and insoluble. Soluble fiber dissolves in water and can help lower blood glucose levels by slowing the absorption of sugar. Foods rich in soluble fiber include oats, beans, lentils, fruits, and some vegetables. Insoluble fiber, on the other hand, does not dissolve in water and aids in digestion by adding bulk to the stool, which helps prevent constipation—a common issue among seniors. Whole grains, nuts, and seeds are excellent sources of insoluble fiber. A balanced intake of both types of fiber is essential for optimal health.

For seniors managing diabetes, fiber-rich foods can also support heart health. High-fiber diets have been linked to lower cholesterol levels, which is particularly important since individuals with diabetes are at a higher risk for cardiovascular disease. Consuming foods high in fiber can help to reduce overall cholesterol and promote better blood pressure levels. This is particularly beneficial for seniors, who may already be dealing with heart-related health issues or medications that can impact heart health.

Incorporating more fiber into the diet can be done gradually to avoid gastrointestinal discomfort. Seniors should aim to increase their fiber intake through whole foods rather than supplements, as whole foods also provide essential vitamins and minerals. Simple changes like choosing whole grain bread instead of white bread, adding beans to salads and soups, and snacking on fruits and vegetables can significantly boost fiber intake. It is advisable for seniors to drink plenty of water when increasing fiber, as this helps prevent any digestive issues.

Finally, the role of fiber extends beyond just blood sugar control and digestive health; it can enhance overall well-being. Many seniors find that higher fiber foods provide sustained energy levels, improving their ability to engage in daily activities. By making fiber a priority in their diets, seniors can contribute to better health outcomes, increased vitality, and a higher quality of life. Emphasizing fiber-rich choices is a practical and effective strategy for managing diabetes and maintaining good health as one ages.

Healthy Fats vs. Unhealthy Fats

Understanding the distinction between healthy and unhealthy fats is crucial for diabetic seniors striving to maintain optimal health. Fats are an essential nutrient that provides energy, supports cell growth, and aids in the absorption of certain vitamins. However, not all fats are created equal. Healthy fats, primarily found in plant sources and certain fish, can support heart health and improve insulin sensitivity. In contrast, unhealthy fats, often found in processed foods and animal products, can exacerbate health issues and increase the risk of complications associated with diabetes.

Healthy fats include monounsaturated and polyunsaturated fats, which are beneficial for maintaining good health. Monounsaturated fats, found in foods such as avocados, olive oil, and nuts, can help lower bad cholesterol levels and reduce the risk of heart disease. Polyunsaturated fats, which include omega-3 and omega-6 fatty acids, are vital for brain function and can be found in fatty fish like salmon, walnuts, and flaxseeds. Incorporating these fats into a balanced diet can contribute to better overall health and potentially improve blood sugar control.

On the other hand, unhealthy fats primarily consist of trans fats and saturated fats. Trans fats, often present in processed and fried foods, are known to raise bad cholesterol levels and lower good cholesterol levels, increasing the risk of heart disease. Saturated fats, commonly found in red meat, full-fat dairy products, and certain oils, can also negatively impact heart health when consumed in excess. For diabetic seniors, managing the intake of these fats is essential, as they can lead to complications such as cardiovascular disease, which is a common concern for individuals with diabetes.

To make healthier choices, it is important for diabetic seniors to read food labels carefully. Foods that contain partially hydrogenated oils are likely to contain trans fats, which should be avoided. Instead, selecting whole, unprocessed foods that are rich in healthy fats can enhance dietary quality. Cooking with olive oil, snacking on nuts, and including fatty fish in meals are simple ways to incorporate healthy fats while minimizing unhealthy options. This approach can help diabetic seniors better manage their weight and blood sugar levels.

In conclusion, understanding the difference between healthy and unhealthy fats is vital for diabetic seniors aiming to live well. By focusing on the inclusion of healthy fats while limiting unhealthy fats, individuals can foster better health outcomes and enhance their quality of life. Making informed dietary choices can help mitigate the risks associated with diabetes and promote overall well-being, allowing seniors to enjoy a vibrant and active lifestyle.

Understanding Portion Sizes

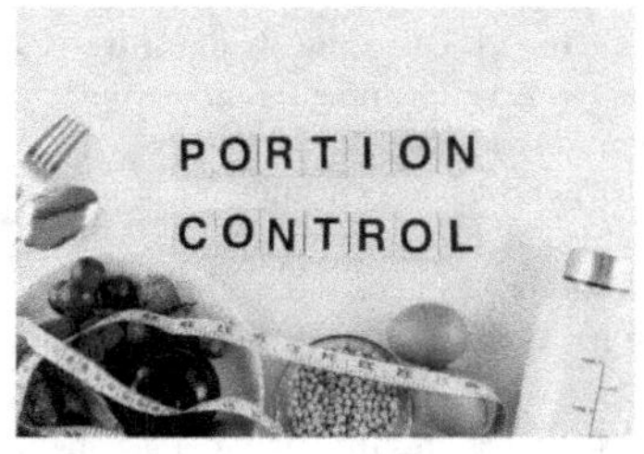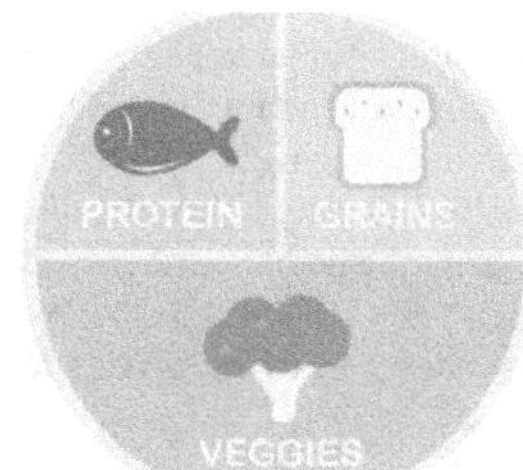

Understanding portion sizes is a crucial aspect of managing diabetes, particularly for seniors who may be navigating various health challenges. Portion sizes refer to the amount of food served in one sitting, and understanding these can help individuals make informed choices that promote better blood sugar control. For seniors, who may have different nutritional needs or appetite levels, recognizing appropriate portion sizes can enhance their overall well-being while preventing complications associated with diabetes.

One effective way to visualize portion sizes is by using everyday items as reference points. For example, a serving of cooked pasta or rice should be roughly the size of a tennis ball, while a serving of protein, such as meat or fish, should be about the size of a deck of cards. Vegetables can be more generous, with a serving typically being about the size of two cupped hands. This method not only simplifies the process of measuring food but also helps seniors avoid the pitfalls of portion distortion that can occur with larger plates and serving sizes commonly found in restaurants or pre-packaged meals.

In addition to visual aids, it's important to understand the concept of carbohydrates, as they play a significant role in blood sugar management. For those with diabetes, monitoring carbohydrate intake is essential, and portion sizes can vary based on individual dietary needs. For example, one carbohydrate serving is typically equivalent to 15 grams of carbs, which can be found in one slice of bread, half a cup of cooked grains, or a medium piece of fruit. By familiarizing themselves with these measurements, seniors can better plan their meals and snacks, ensuring they meet their carbohydrate goals without overindulging.

Seniors should also consider the importance of balance when it comes to portion sizes. A well-rounded meal should include a variety of food groups, such as lean proteins, whole grains, healthy fats, and plenty of vegetables. By incorporating a mix of these elements in appropriate portions, seniors can enjoy a satisfying meal that provides essential nutrients while keeping blood sugar levels stable. Preparing meals at home allows for greater control over portion sizes, making it easier to adhere to dietary guidelines.

Finally, portion sizes can be modified based on individual activity levels, health conditions, and personal preferences. It's essential for seniors to listen to their bodies and adjust their servings accordingly. Keeping a food diary can be a helpful tool in this process, allowing individuals to track their intake and identify patterns over time. By understanding and applying the principles of portion sizes, diabetic seniors can take significant steps toward maintaining their health, improving their quality of life, and managing their diabetes effectively.

Chapter 4: Exercise and Physical Activity
Benefits of Regular Exercise

Regular exercise offers numerous benefits for seniors living with diabetes, significantly enhancing both physical and mental health. One of the primary advantages is improved blood sugar control. Engaging in physical activity helps muscles use glucose more effectively, which can lead to lower blood sugar levels. Exercise boosts insulin sensitivity, allowing the body to utilize insulin more efficiently. This is particularly important for seniors, as maintaining stable blood sugar levels can prevent complications associated with diabetes, such as neuropathy and cardiovascular issues.

In addition to blood sugar management, regular exercise contributes to weight management. Many seniors find it challenging to maintain a healthy weight, which is crucial for diabetes management. Physical activity helps burn calories and build lean muscle mass, which can increase metabolism. Even moderate activities like walking or swimming can support weight loss or maintenance efforts. A healthy weight can significantly reduce the risk of diabetes-related complications and enhance overall well-being.

Exercise also plays a vital role in improving cardiovascular health, which is especially important for seniors with diabetes. People with diabetes are at a higher risk for heart disease, making cardiovascular health a priority. Regular physical activity strengthens the heart, improves circulation, and lowers blood pressure and cholesterol levels. Engaging in aerobic exercises, such as brisk walking or cycling, can lead to substantial cardiovascular benefits, reducing the risk of heart attacks and strokes.

Mental health is another critical area positively impacted by regular exercise. Seniors often face challenges such as depression and anxiety, which can be exacerbated by the stresses of managing diabetes. Physical activity releases endorphins, known as "feel-good" hormones, which can improve mood and reduce feelings of anxiety. Furthermore, exercise can enhance cognitive function, helping seniors maintain mental sharpness and reduce the risk of cognitive decline. Activities that involve coordination and balance, such as tai chi or yoga, can also promote mindfulness and relaxation.

Lastly, regular exercise fosters a sense of community and social interaction, which is beneficial for emotional health. Many seniors find companionship and support in group exercise classes or walking clubs. These social connections can combat feelings of isolation and loneliness, often experienced by older adults. By participating in physical activities with others, seniors can build friendships, share experiences, and encourage each other in their fitness journeys. Overall,

incorporating regular exercise into daily routines can significantly improve the quality of life for diabetic seniors, helping them lead healthier, happier lives.

Types of Exercise for Seniors

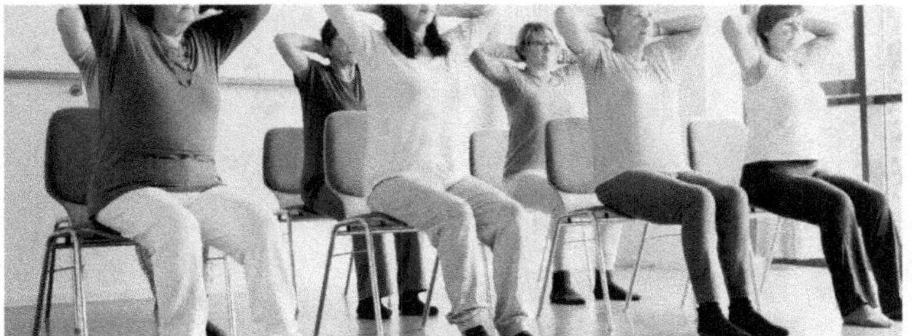

Exercise plays a crucial role in managing diabetes, particularly for seniors. Engaging in regular physical activity can help maintain a healthy weight, improve blood sugar control, and reduce the risk of complications associated with diabetes. Understanding the various types of exercise suitable for seniors can empower individuals to incorporate movement into their daily routine, fostering a healthier lifestyle and enhancing overall well-being.

Aerobic exercise is one of the most beneficial forms of physical activity for seniors with diabetes. This type of exercise includes activities that increase the heart rate and improve cardiovascular health, such as walking, swimming, and cycling. Aerobic exercises can enhance insulin sensitivity and help regulate blood sugar levels, making them particularly advantageous for diabetic individuals. Seniors should aim for at least 150 minutes of moderate-intensity aerobic exercise each week, breaking this down into manageable sessions throughout the week.

Strength training is another essential component of an effective exercise regimen. It helps in building muscle mass, which can deteriorate with age, and boosts metabolism, aiding in weight management. Simple resistance exercises using light weights, resistance bands, or even bodyweight can be performed safely at home or in a gym setting. Seniors should focus on major muscle groups, aiming to incorporate strength training at least twice a week. This not only improves physical strength but also supports joint health and enhances balance, reducing the risk of falls.

Flexibility and balance exercises are vital for seniors, particularly those with diabetes, as they can help prevent injuries and improve overall mobility. Activities such as yoga, tai chi, and stretching routines promote flexibility and enhance balance, which is crucial for maintaining independence. These exercises can also contribute to better relaxation and stress management, further benefiting blood sugar control. Incorporating a few minutes of flexibility and balance exercises into daily routines can yield significant improvements in physical function.

Lastly, incorporating activities that promote social interaction can enhance the exercise experience for seniors. Group classes, community walks, or even gardening can provide both physical activity and social engagement. Such activities not only make exercise more enjoyable but also foster a sense of community and support, which can be particularly beneficial for seniors managing diabetes. By exploring various types of exercise, seniors can create a balanced and enjoyable fitness routine that supports their health and well-being in living well with diabetes.

Creating a Safe Exercise Routine

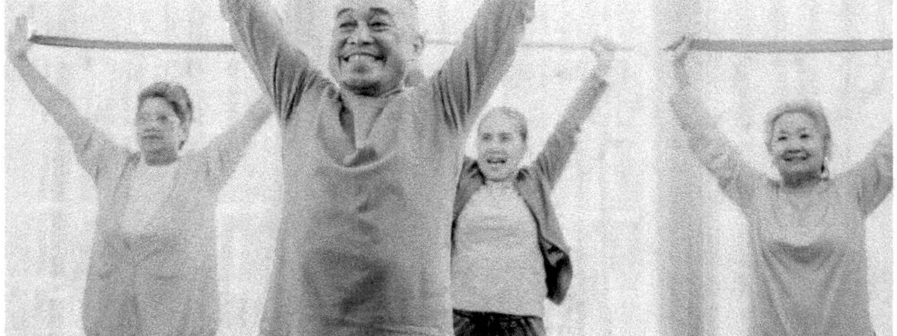

Creating a safe exercise routine is essential for diabetic seniors to manage their condition effectively while enhancing their overall health. Regular physical activity helps regulate blood sugar levels, improve cardiovascular health, and maintain a healthy weight. However, it is crucial for seniors to approach exercise with caution, considering their unique health status and any pre-existing conditions. By taking the right steps, seniors can create a safe and enjoyable exercise routine tailored to their needs.

Before initiating any exercise program, it is important for diabetic seniors to consult with healthcare professionals. A physician can provide personalized recommendations based on individual health conditions, medications, and fitness levels. This consultation may include a comprehensive evaluation, which could highlight any limitations or precautions that should be considered. In addition, a referral to a physical therapist or a certified fitness trainer with experience in senior fitness and diabetes management can be beneficial, ensuring that the exercises chosen are safe and effective.

Once a healthcare provider has approved a fitness regimen, seniors can begin by incorporating low-impact activities into their routine. Walking, swimming, and cycling are excellent options that minimize stress on the joints while promoting cardiovascular fitness. These activities can be performed at a moderate pace, allowing seniors to gradually build endurance without overexerting themselves. It is advisable to start with shorter sessions, around 10 to 15 minutes, and gradually increase the duration as stamina improves.

Monitoring blood sugar levels before, during, and after exercise is crucial for diabetic seniors. Physical activity can affect blood glucose levels in different ways, and being aware of these changes can help prevent both hypoglycemia and hyperglycemia. Seniors should always have a source of fast-acting carbohydrates on hand, such as glucose tablets or juice, to quickly address low blood sugar levels. By creating a structured and informed exercise routine, diabetic seniors can enhance their quality of life, manage their condition, and enjoy the numerous health benefits that regular physical activity offers.

In addition to aerobic exercises, strength training is an important component of a well-rounded fitness routine. Engaging in resistance exercises, such as using light weights or resistance bands, helps maintain muscle mass and supports metabolic health. Seniors should aim for strength training sessions at least two days a week, focusing on major muscle groups. Importantly, proper form and technique should be prioritized to prevent injury, and it may be beneficial to work with a professional initially to ensure exercises are performed safely.

Staying Motivated

Staying motivated is crucial for diabetic seniors as they navigate the challenges of managing their health. Motivation can often fluctuate, especially when facing the daily demands of dietary restrictions, medication management, and the need for regular physical activity. Recognizing this, it's important to develop strategies that can help maintain a consistent level of motivation. This begins with setting attainable goals that align with personal health objectives. By focusing on achievable milestones, seniors can experience a sense of accomplishment that fuels further motivation.

Establishing a routine is another effective way to stay motivated. Consistency can create a sense of normalcy and order in daily life, which is especially beneficial for managing diabetes. Seniors should consider setting specific times for meals, exercise, and medication. Incorporating these activities into a daily schedule can reduce decision fatigue and make it easier to adhere to a healthy lifestyle. Additionally, having a structured routine allows for the tracking of progress, which can be a powerful motivator in itself.

Engagement in social activities can greatly enhance motivation for diabetic seniors. Connecting with others who share similar experiences can provide encouragement and support. This might involve participating in group exercise classes tailored for seniors, joining diabetes support groups, or even sharing healthy cooking sessions with friends or family. The social aspect of these activities not only boosts motivation but also makes the journey toward better health more enjoyable and less isolating.

Celebrating successes, no matter how small, can also play a significant role in maintaining motivation. Recognizing achievements, whether it's sticking to a meal plan for a week or successfully incorporating daily walks, reinforces positive behavior and encourages seniors to continue on their path. Keeping a journal to document these successes can serve as a tangible reminder of progress and dedication. Seniors should also consider rewarding themselves for reaching certain milestones, which can provide additional incentive to stay committed to their health goals.

Finally, it's essential to cultivate a positive mindset when faced with challenges. Diabetes management can sometimes feel overwhelming, but maintaining a hopeful and proactive attitude can make a significant difference. Engaging in mindfulness practices, such as meditation or gentle yoga, can help reduce stress and improve overall well-being. Furthermore, seeking guidance from healthcare professionals can empower seniors with the knowledge and resources needed to make informed decisions about their health. By fostering a supportive environment and focusing on the positives, seniors can enhance their motivation and lead fulfilling lives while managing diabetes.

Chapter 5: Monitoring Blood Sugar Levels
Understanding Blood Sugar Readings

Blood sugar readings are essential for managing diabetes, especially for seniors who may face unique health challenges. Understanding these readings can empower individuals to make informed decisions about their diet, medication, and lifestyle. Blood sugar levels are typically measured in milligrams per deciliter (mg/dL), and they can fluctuate throughout the day based on various factors such as food intake, physical activity, stress, and medication. Familiarizing oneself with the normal ranges and how to interpret these readings is crucial for effective diabetes management.

For most adults, a normal fasting blood sugar level is between 70 and 99 mg/dL. After eating, blood sugar levels can rise, but they should generally remain below 140 mg/dL two hours post-meal. Consistently higher readings can indicate prediabetes or diabetes, while lower readings may suggest hypoglycemia, a condition that can be especially dangerous for seniors. It is vital to understand that individual targets may vary based on personal health conditions, medications, and the advice of healthcare providers. Regular consultation with a doctor or diabetes educator can help seniors establish their specific blood sugar goals.

Seniors should also be aware of the importance of monitoring their blood sugar levels regularly. Self-monitoring can help detect patterns and identify how different foods, activities, and medications influence blood sugar. Keeping a log of readings can provide valuable insight and assist healthcare providers in making necessary adjustments to treatment plans. Many modern blood glucose meters allow users to track their readings easily, and some even connect to smartphone apps, making it simpler to share data with healthcare professionals.

In addition to monitoring, understanding the factors that affect blood sugar levels is crucial. Diet plays a significant role; foods high in carbohydrates can cause blood sugar spikes, while fiber-rich foods can help regulate levels. Seniors should focus on balanced meals that include lean proteins, healthy fats, and whole grains. Physical activity is another vital factor; even moderate exercise, like walking or gardening, can help control blood sugar levels. Seniors should consult their healthcare team to create a tailored plan that incorporates both diet and exercise.

Finally, it is essential for seniors to recognize the signs of blood sugar fluctuations. Symptoms of high blood sugar may include increased thirst, frequent urination, and fatigue, while low blood sugar can result in shakiness, confusion, and dizziness. Being aware of these symptoms allows for timely intervention, whether it's adjusting medication, consuming a quick source of sugar, or seeking medical attention. By understanding blood sugar readings and their implications,

seniors can take proactive steps toward managing their diabetes effectively and living healthier, more fulfilling lives.

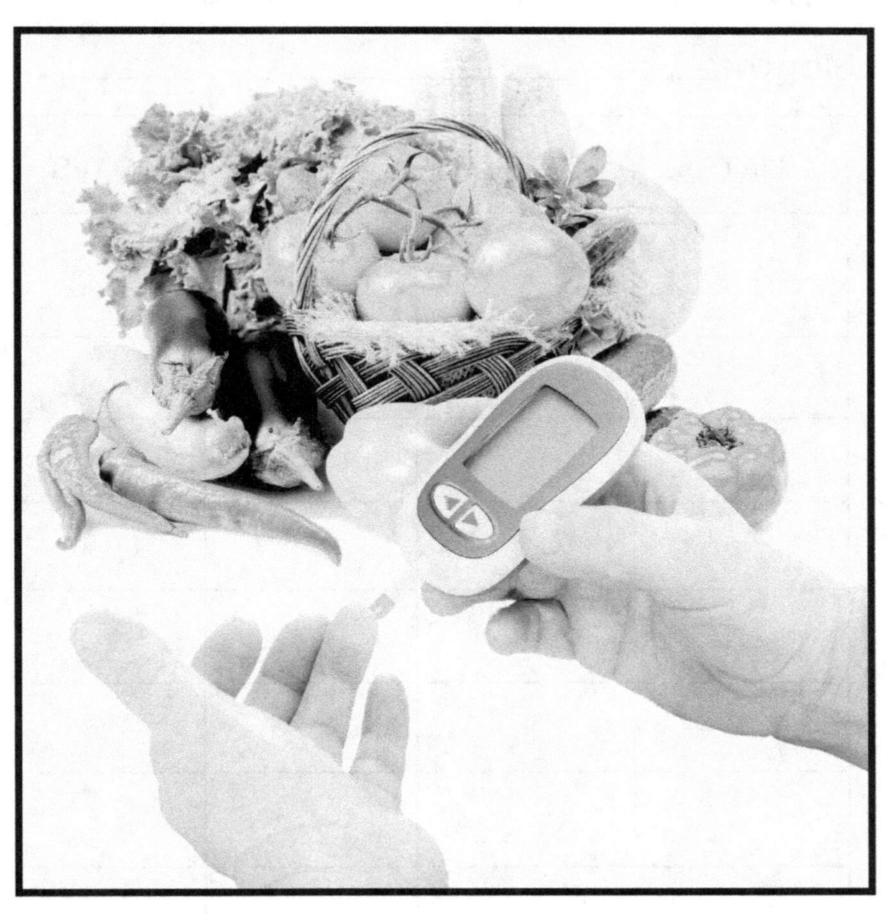

Keep monitoring your blood sugar and keep a log for your doctor

BLOOD SUGAR TRACKER

Month:_______________________________________

DATE	LEVEL	TIME	NOTES

Patient's name:_______________________________

BLOOD SUGAR TRACKER

Month:________________________________

DATE	LEVEL	TIME	NOTES

Patient's name:________________________________

BLOOD SUGAR TRACKER

Month:_____________________________________

DATE	LEVEL	TIME	NOTES

Patient's name:_____________________________

BLOOD SUGAR TRACKER

Month:______________________________________

DATE	LEVEL	TIME	NOTES

Patient's name:______________________________________

Keeping a Blood Sugar Log

Keeping a blood sugar log is an essential practice for managing diabetes, especially for seniors who may face unique challenges in their daily routines. A blood sugar log serves as a record of your glucose levels over time, helping you and your healthcare team identify patterns and make informed decisions about your treatment. This log can be an invaluable tool in understanding how various factors such as food, exercise, medications, and stress impact your blood sugar levels.

To start a blood sugar log, choose a format that works best for you, whether it's a handwritten notebook, a digital app, or a spreadsheet. Consistency is key, so make it a habit to record your blood sugar readings at the same times each day. Many seniors find it helpful to measure their levels before and after meals, as well as before bedtime. This routine not only provides a clearer picture of how your body responds to different foods and activities but also allows you to detect trends that may require attention.

In addition to recording blood sugar readings, it's important to document other relevant information in your log. Include details such as the time of day, what you ate, your physical activity, and any medications taken. Noting how you feel at the time of each reading can also provide insight into your overall well-being. For instance, if you notice a pattern of high glucose levels after certain meals, you may need to reconsider your food choices or portion sizes. This comprehensive approach will empower you to take charge of your health.

Reviewing your blood sugar log regularly is a crucial step in diabetes management. Set aside time each week or month to analyze the data, looking for any significant fluctuations or patterns. If you notice consistent highs or lows, consider discussing these findings with your healthcare provider. They can help you adjust your treatment plan, whether that involves changing medications, modifying your diet, or increasing physical activity. This proactive approach can lead to better blood sugar control and overall health.

Finally, sharing your blood sugar log with family members or caregivers can enhance your support system. They can help remind you to check your levels and assist in interpreting the data. Involving loved ones in your diabetes management can foster a sense of accountability and encouragement, making it easier to stick to healthy habits. By keeping a detailed blood sugar log, you are taking an important step toward living well with diabetes and maintaining a healthier, more active lifestyle.

Recognizing and Responding to High and Low Levels

Recognizing and responding to high and low blood sugar levels is crucial for managing diabetes effectively. Seniors, in particular, may experience fluctuations in their blood glucose levels due to various factors, including changes in diet, physical activity, medications, and overall health conditions. It is essential for diabetic seniors to familiarize themselves with the symptoms of both hyperglycemia (high blood sugar) and hypoglycemia (low blood sugar) to take timely actions and prevent complications.

Hyperglycemia can manifest through various symptoms, including excessive thirst, frequent urination, fatigue, and blurred vision. In some cases it may lead to more severe conditions such as diabetic ketoacidosis if not addressed promptly. Seniors should monitor their blood sugar levels regularly, especially after meals, and be aware of their personal triggers. Keeping a log of blood sugar readings can help identify patterns, allowing for better management of diet and medication schedules.

On the other hand, recognizing the signs of hypoglycemia is equally important. Symptoms such as shakiness, sweating, confusion, irritability, and dizziness can indicate dangerously low blood sugar levels. Seniors may also experience a sudden hunger pang or a racing heartbeat. It is vital to act quickly in these situations by consuming fast-acting carbohydrates, such as glucose tablets or sugary drinks, to raise blood sugar levels promptly. Having a source of quick sugar readily available is a practical step that can prevent serious complications.

Maintaining open communication with healthcare providers is essential for seniors managing diabetes. Regular check-ups can ensure that medications are appropriately adjusted according to the individual's changing needs. Senior diabetics should also work with their healthcare team to create a personalized action plan for both high and low blood sugar episodes. This may include specific instructions on when to use insulin, how to adjust meals or snacks, and what to do in the event of severe hypoglycemia.

In addition to monitoring blood sugar levels and adhering to medication regimens, lifestyle changes play a significant role in managing diabetes. Engaging in regular physical activity, following a balanced diet, and ensuring adequate hydration can help stabilize blood sugar levels. Seniors should also consider the impact of stress and illness on their diabetes management. By being proactive and informed, diabetic seniors can lead healthier lives while effectively recognizing and responding to the fluctuations in their blood sugar levels.

Chapter 6: Managing Medications
Types of Diabetes Medications

Diabetes medications play a crucial role in managing blood sugar levels and preventing complications associated with the disease. For seniors, understanding the different types of diabetes medications is essential for making informed choices about their health. The primary classes of medications include insulin, oral hypoglycemics, and non-insulin injectables, each with unique mechanisms of action, benefits, and potential side effects.

Insulin is a hormone that helps regulate blood sugar levels by facilitating the uptake of glucose into cells. For many seniors with Type 1 diabetes, insulin is a necessary treatment, as their bodies do not produce it. In Type 2 diabetes, insulin may be prescribed when other medications are insufficient to control blood sugar. Insulin can be administered through injections or insulin pumps, and it is important for seniors to monitor their blood sugar levels closely to avoid hypoglycemia, which can be particularly dangerous.

Oral hypoglycemics are another common type of medication for managing Type 2 diabetes. These medications work in various ways to lower blood sugar levels. Sulfonylureas stimulate the pancreas to produce more insulin, while biguanides, such as metformin, reduce glucose production in the liver and improve insulin sensitivity. Other classes, like DPP-4 inhibitors and SGLT2 inhibitors, have distinct mechanisms and may offer additional benefits, such as weight loss or cardiovascular protection. Seniors should consult their healthcare providers to determine which oral medications are most suitable for their individual health profiles.

Non-insulin injectables, such as GLP-1 receptor agonists, are another option for seniors with Type 2 diabetes. These medications mimic the action of incretin hormones, which help regulate insulin secretion and decrease appetite. They can lead to weight loss and improved blood sugar control. However, they may also cause gastrointestinal side effects, which seniors should be aware of. Understanding how these medications work can empower seniors to make choices that align with their lifestyle and health goals.

When considering diabetes medications, seniors must take into account their overall health, existing medical conditions, and potential interactions with other medications. Regular consultations with healthcare professionals are vital in managing diabetes effectively. By staying informed about the various types of medications available and their respective benefits and

risks, seniors can take proactive steps toward living well with diabetes, leading to a healthier and more fulfilling life.

Importance of Adherence to Medication

Adherence to medication is a critical component of managing diabetes, especially for seniors who may face unique challenges in their healthcare journey. Medications prescribed for diabetes, such as insulin and oral hypoglycemics, play a vital role in controlling blood sugar levels and preventing complications. For seniors, who often have multiple health issues and take various medications, understanding the importance of adherence becomes paramount. Consistently following the prescribed medication regimen helps maintain stable blood glucose levels, reducing the risk of both short-term and long-term complications associated with diabetes.

One of the primary reasons adherence to medication is crucial is that it helps prevent complications such as cardiovascular disease, kidney failure, and neuropathy. Seniors with diabetes are already at a higher risk for these conditions, and inconsistent medication can exacerbate these risks. Regularly taking medications as directed can help mitigate these dangers, ensuring that seniors maintain their health and quality of life. Additionally, adhering to medication can reduce the likelihood of emergency medical situations, which can be particularly challenging for seniors who may have mobility issues or limited access to immediate care.

Furthermore, adhering to medication can enhance the overall effectiveness of diabetes management strategies. Medications work best when combined with lifestyle changes such as a balanced diet and regular exercise. When seniors take their medications as prescribed, they are more likely to experience improved blood sugar control, which can lead to better overall health outcomes. This synergy between medication adherence and lifestyle changes is essential for achieving and maintaining optimal diabetes management, allowing seniors to enjoy their daily activities with greater ease and comfort.

Seniors may encounter various barriers to medication adherence, including cognitive decline, vision problems, and complex medication regimens. It is essential for caregivers and healthcare providers to recognize these challenges and offer support tailored to each senior's needs. Simple strategies, such as using pill organizers, setting reminders, or simplifying medication schedules, can significantly improve adherence. Additionally, open communication between seniors and their healthcare team can help ensure that any concerns or difficulties related to medication are addressed promptly, fostering a cooperative approach to diabetes management.

In conclusion, the importance of adherence to medication in managing diabetes among seniors cannot be overstated. By consistently following their prescribed medication regimens, seniors can significantly reduce the risk of complications, enhance the effectiveness of their diabetes management strategies, and ultimately improve their quality of life. Awareness of the challenges

that may hinder adherence and the implementation of supportive measures can empower seniors to take control of their health, enabling them to live well with diabetes.

Communicating with Healthcare Providers

Effective communication with healthcare providers is essential for diabetic seniors to manage their condition and maintain a healthy lifestyle. This includes understanding medication regimens, dietary restrictions, and the importance of regular check-ups. Seniors should approach their healthcare appointments prepared, armed with questions and a clear understanding of their health status. This proactive approach not only aids in receiving tailored treatment but also fosters a collaborative relationship with healthcare professionals.

Seniors should be aware of the specific aspects of their diabetes that need to be communicated during consultations. This includes blood sugar levels, any recent changes in health, and how diabetes is affecting their daily life. Keeping a log of symptoms, medication side effects, and dietary habits can provide valuable insights for healthcare providers. It is crucial to be honest about lifestyle choices and challenges faced in managing diabetes, as this will enable providers to offer more personalized advice and support.

In addition to verbal communication, seniors can benefit from utilizing written materials. Bringing along a list of medications, allergies, and any other relevant health conditions can help streamline discussions. Seniors should also consider asking for written instructions regarding treatment plans or dietary recommendations. This documentation can serve as a helpful reference at home, reinforcing what was discussed during the appointment and ensuring adherence to medical advice.

Seniors are encouraged to ask questions if they do not understand something. Healthcare providers appreciate when patients seek clarification, as it indicates engagement in their own health management. Common questions may include inquiries about the implications of blood sugar readings, potential side effects of medications, or alternative therapies. Understanding the answers to these questions can significantly enhance a senior's ability to manage their diabetes effectively.

Finally, maintaining an open line of communication with healthcare providers between appointments is vital. Seniors should feel empowered to reach out with concerns or changes in their health status. Many healthcare systems offer patient portals where seniors can send messages or access test results conveniently. By staying in touch and expressing concerns, diabetic seniors can ensure that they are receiving ongoing support and adjustments to their care plan as needed. This proactive communication fosters a sense of partnership in the management of their diabetes, ultimately leading to better health outcomes.

Understanding Side Effects

Understanding side effects is crucial for diabetic seniors who are managing their health. As individuals age, their bodies undergo numerous changes that can affect how medications work and how they interact with various health conditions. Side effects can arise from diabetes medications, dietary changes, or even lifestyle adjustments made to manage the condition. It is essential for seniors to be aware of these potential effects to make informed decisions about their treatment and lifestyle.

The most common side effects associated with diabetes medications include gastrointestinal issues, hypoglycemia, and weight gain. Gastrointestinal problems, such as nausea or diarrhea, can occur with certain oral medications. Hypoglycemia, or low blood sugar, is particularly concerning for seniors, as it can lead to confusion, dizziness, and even loss of consciousness. Weight gain can also be a side effect of some diabetes medications, which may complicate blood sugar management. Understanding these potential side effects can help seniors recognize symptoms early and communicate effectively with their healthcare providers.

Aside from medications, dietary changes can also lead to side effects. For instance, adopting a low-carbohydrate or ketogenic diet may result in initial fatigue or headaches as the body adjusts to a new source of energy. Additionally, changes in fiber intake can cause digestive disturbances. It is important for seniors to approach dietary changes gradually and to monitor their bodies' responses to new foods. Keeping a food diary could be beneficial in identifying any adverse reactions to specific dietary choices.

Exercise is another critical component of diabetes management that can come with its own set of side effects. While regular physical activity is vital for maintaining blood sugar levels, seniors may experience soreness, fatigue, or even injury if they push themselves too hard. It is essential for seniors to engage in physical activity that is appropriate for their fitness level and to consult with healthcare professionals before starting new exercise routines. Understanding one's limits can help prevent negative side effects while still reaping the benefits of a more active lifestyle.

In conclusion, awareness of side effects is a vital part of diabetes management for seniors. By understanding the potential side effects of medications, dietary changes, and exercise, seniors can better navigate their health journey. Open communication with healthcare providers about any experienced side effects can lead to adjustments in treatment plans, ultimately fostering a more successful and healthy management of diabetes. Being informed and proactive can help seniors maintain their well-being and enjoy a higher quality of life.

Chapter 7: Complications and Preventative Care

Common Diabetes Complications

Diabetes can lead to a range of complications that affect various parts of the body, particularly in seniors. Understanding these complications is crucial for managing diabetes effectively and maintaining a high quality of life. The most common complications include cardiovascular diseases, nerve damage, kidney damage, eye problems, and foot issues. Each of these complications can have a significant impact on health and wellbeing, making early detection and intervention essential.

Cardiovascular diseases are among the most serious complications associated with diabetes. Seniors with diabetes are at a higher risk for heart disease, stroke, and high blood pressure. The damage caused by elevated blood sugar levels can lead to atherosclerosis, a condition where the arteries become narrowed and hardened due to plaque build-up. This increases the likelihood of heart attacks and strokes, emphasizing the importance of regular cardiovascular check-ups and lifestyle modifications, such as a heart-healthy diet and regular physical activity.

Nerve damage, known as diabetic neuropathy, is another common complication that affects many seniors with diabetes. High blood sugar levels can harm the nerves, particularly in the feet and legs, leading to symptoms such as numbness, tingling, and pain. This can affect balance and mobility, increasing the risk of falls. Seniors should be vigilant about monitoring their foot health, as nerve damage can also lead to unnoticed injuries or infections, which can become serious if not treated promptly.

Kidney damage, or diabetic nephropathy, is a significant concern for seniors living with diabetes. The kidneys play a crucial role in filtering waste from the blood, and diabetes can impair this function over time. Regular kidney function tests are important for early detection of any issues. Lifestyle choices, such as managing blood pressure and blood sugar levels, along with staying hydrated and avoiding excessive protein intake, can help protect kidney health.

Eye problems, including diabetic retinopathy, cataracts, and glaucoma, are also prevalent among seniors with diabetes. Elevated blood sugar levels can damage the blood vessels in the retina, leading to vision loss if not addressed. Regular eye examinations are essential for early detection and treatment of these conditions. Seniors should prioritize eye care as part of their diabetes management plan to preserve their vision and overall quality of life.

Foot issues can arise due to a combination of nerve damage and poor circulation, both of which are common in seniors with diabetes. This can lead to ulcers, infections, and in severe cases,

Managing Foot Health

Foot health is a crucial aspect of diabetes management, particularly for seniors. Diabetes can lead to neuropathy, a condition that causes nerve damage and can reduce sensation in the feet. This loss of feeling makes it difficult to detect injuries, blisters, or infections. Regularly inspecting your feet for any signs of cuts, blisters, or changes in color is essential. Seniors should make it a habit to check their feet daily, using a mirror if necessary, to ensure they do not overlook any potential issues.

Proper footwear is another vital component of maintaining foot health. Footwear that fits well and offers adequate support can help prevent injuries and discomfort. Seniors should choose shoes that provide a good fit, cushioning, and arch support. Avoiding tight shoes or those with pointed toes can also help reduce the risk of foot problems. Additionally, consider using diabetic socks, which are designed to reduce pressure points and wick moisture away from the skin, thus minimizing the risk of blisters and fungal infections.

Moisturizing the feet is an important practice that many seniors may overlook. Dry skin can lead to cracking, which increases the risk of infection. Applying a gentle, fragrance-free moisturizer to the tops and bottoms of the feet can help maintain skin integrity. However, it is essential to avoid applying lotion between the toes, as moisture accumulation in that area can lead to fungal infections. Regularly caring for the skin on your feet can contribute significantly to overall foot health.

Regular visits to a healthcare provider for foot examinations are crucial for diabetic seniors. A podiatrist can assess foot health, provide professional cleaning, and identify any early signs of complications. Seniors should inform their healthcare providers about any changes or concerns they notice regarding their foot health. Early intervention can prevent serious complications, including infections that may require hospitalization or surgery.

Incorporating foot exercises into your daily routine can also enhance foot health. Simple exercises such as toe lifts, ankle rotations, and stretching can improve circulation and maintain flexibility. Engaging in regular physical activity, such as walking, can promote overall circulation, which is especially beneficial for individuals with diabetes. By taking these proactive steps in managing foot health, seniors can significantly reduce their risk of complications and maintain mobility and independence.

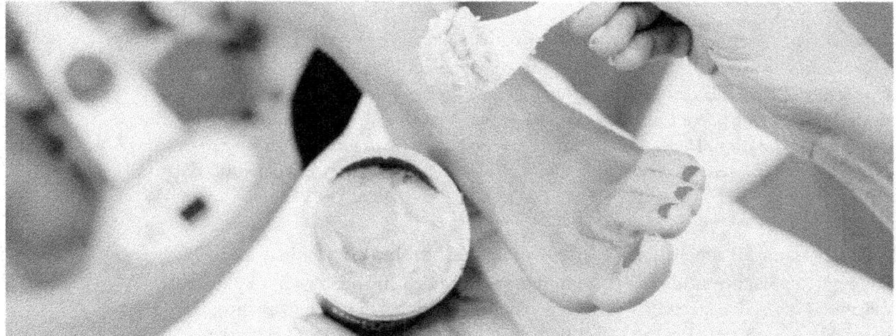

Chapter 8: Emotional and Mental Well-being
The Psychological Impact of Diabetes

The psychological impact of diabetes can be profound, particularly for seniors who may already be navigating other health challenges. Living with diabetes often requires constant attention to dietary choices, medication management, and monitoring blood sugar levels. This ongoing need

for vigilance can lead to feelings of anxiety and stress, as seniors may worry about the potential complications associated with poorly managed diabetes. Understanding these psychological effects is crucial for seniors to develop strategies that support their mental health alongside their physical well-being.

Many seniors with diabetes experience a sense of loss related to their former lifestyles. The need for dietary restrictions and changes in daily routines can evoke feelings of frustration and sadness. This sense of loss can manifest as a decreased appetite or reluctance to engage in social activities, especially those centered around food. It is important for seniors to acknowledge these feelings and to find new ways to enjoy meals and social gatherings that align with their health goals. By focusing on the positive aspects of their dietary changes, seniors can foster a healthier relationship with food.

Fear of complications is another significant psychological impact of diabetes. Seniors may feel overwhelmed by the potential for serious health issues, such as heart disease, nerve damage, or vision problems. This fear can lead to a heightened state of anxiety, making it difficult to manage their condition effectively. Education plays a vital role in alleviating these fears. Understanding diabetes and its management can empower seniors to take control of their health, reducing anxiety and promoting a more positive outlook on living with the condition.

Social isolation is a common concern for seniors with diabetes. The need for careful meal planning and monitoring can make it challenging to engage in social activities. Seniors may feel embarrassed or anxious about their dietary needs, leading them to withdraw from social situations. Encouraging participation in diabetes support groups or community activities can help combat this isolation. These social connections provide a platform for sharing experiences and strategies, helping seniors feel less alone in their journey and fostering a sense of belonging.

Finally, it is essential for seniors to prioritize their mental health as part of their overall diabetes management. Regular physical activity, mindfulness practices, and hobbies can significantly improve mood and reduce feelings of stress. Seeking professional help, whether through therapy or counseling, can also provide valuable support for those struggling with the psychological aspects of diabetes. By adopting a comprehensive approach that includes both physical and mental health, seniors can enhance their quality of life and live well with diabetes.

Stress Management Techniques

Stress management is an essential aspect of maintaining overall health, especially for seniors living with diabetes. The relationship between stress and diabetes is complex; stress can lead to hormonal changes that affect blood sugar levels, making it crucial to implement effective stress

management techniques. By managing stress, seniors can improve their emotional well-being and potentially stabilize their glucose levels, leading to better health outcomes.

One effective technique for managing stress is mindfulness meditation. This practice involves focusing on the present moment, acknowledging thoughts and feelings without judgment. Seniors can start with just a few minutes each day, gradually increasing the duration as they become more comfortable. Mindfulness meditation can help reduce anxiety and increase awareness of bodily sensations, which is particularly beneficial for those monitoring their blood sugar levels. Incorporating this technique into daily routines can foster a sense of calm and clarity.

Physical activity is another powerful stress reliever that can significantly benefit diabetic seniors. Engaging in regular exercise, such as walking, swimming, or gentle yoga, not only helps to reduce stress but also promotes better blood sugar control and overall physical health. Exercise releases endorphins, the body's natural mood elevators, which can enhance feelings of well-being. Seniors should aim for at least 150 minutes of moderate-intensity aerobic activity each week, as recommended by health professionals, while also considering activities that they enjoy to maintain motivation.

Social connections also play a vital role in stress management. Maintaining relationships with family, friends, and community members can provide emotional support and reduce feelings of loneliness, which can exacerbate stress. Seniors can engage in social activities such as joining clubs, participating in group exercise classes, or volunteering in their communities. These interactions can create a sense of belonging and purpose, leading to lower stress levels and improved mental health.

Lastly, establishing a routine can help diabetic seniors manage stress more effectively. A structured daily schedule that includes time for meals, medication, physical activity, and relaxation can create a sense of stability. Seniors should prioritize sleep and ensure they are getting enough rest, as fatigue can heighten stress levels. By incorporating these stress management techniques into their daily lives, seniors with diabetes can enhance their quality of life, making it easier to navigate the challenges of living with this condition.

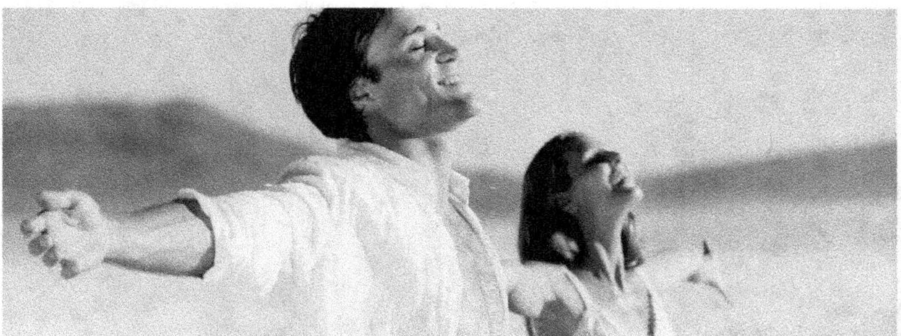

Building a Support Network

Building a support network is essential for diabetic seniors who seek to manage their condition effectively. A well-established support network can provide emotional encouragement, practical advice, and valuable resources that can enhance one's quality of life. This network can include

family members, friends, healthcare professionals, and support groups specifically tailored for individuals living with diabetes. Each component of the network plays a vital role in helping seniors navigate the complexities of diabetes management and encourages a sense of community and belonging.

Family members often serve as the first line of support. They can assist with daily tasks such as meal preparation, exercise routines, and medication management. Engaging family members in discussions about diabetes can increase their understanding of the condition and its challenges. This awareness enables them to offer more meaningful support and helps create an environment that fosters healthy habits. Seniors should communicate openly with their loved ones about their needs and preferences, ensuring that their support is aligned with their lifestyle choices.

Healthcare professionals are another critical element of a robust support network. Regular consultations with doctors, nurses, and dietitians provide seniors with expert guidance tailored to their specific health needs. These professionals can offer customized advice on managing blood sugar levels, creating meal plans, and developing exercise regimens. They can also facilitate connections with other healthcare resources, such as diabetes educators and specialists, who can provide additional insights and support. Building a trusting relationship with these professionals is crucial, as it encourages consistent follow-up and proactive management of diabetes.

Support groups specifically designed for diabetic seniors can be incredibly beneficial. These groups provide a safe space for individuals to share experiences, challenges, and successes. Interacting with peers who understand the unique hurdles of living with diabetes can foster a sense of camaraderie and reduce feelings of isolation. Participants can learn new coping strategies and gain motivation from one another, making it easier to adhere to lifestyle changes. Many communities offer local support groups, while online forums can also serve as platforms for connection and information exchange.

In conclusion, building a support network is a vital step for seniors managing diabetes. By engaging family members, healthcare professionals, and peer support groups, individuals can create a comprehensive system of assistance that addresses both their emotional and practical needs. This network not only enhances diabetes management but also contributes to an improved overall sense of well-being. By actively nurturing these relationships, diabetic seniors can empower themselves to live healthier and more fulfilling lives.

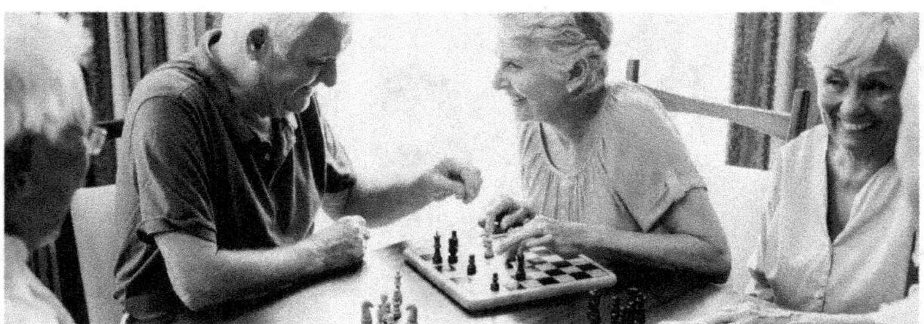

Resources for Mental Health

Mental health is an essential component of overall well-being, especially for seniors managing diabetes. Understanding the connection between mental and physical health can empower

diabetic seniors to seek out the resources they need. Various organizations and online platforms provide valuable information and support tailored to the unique challenges faced by seniors living with diabetes. These resources can help individuals navigate their mental health while maintaining their physical health.

One prominent resource is the National Institute of Mental Health, which offers comprehensive information on mental health conditions, treatment options, and coping strategies. Their website includes fact sheets and research findings specifically addressing the mental health concerns prevalent among older adults. Additionally, they provide guidance on recognizing the signs of depression and anxiety, which can be exacerbated by chronic illnesses like diabetes. Accessing this information can help seniors become more aware of their mental health needs and encourage them to seek appropriate support.

Local community centers often provide programs specifically designed for seniors, including support groups and workshops that focus on mental well-being. Engaging in these community-based activities can foster social connections, reduce feelings of isolation, and promote a sense of belonging. Many centers also collaborate with mental health professionals, allowing for workshops that teach coping strategies and stress management techniques. Participating in such programs can not only enhance mental health but also encourage seniors to maintain a healthy lifestyle, which is crucial for diabetes management.

Online therapy and counseling services have become increasingly popular, especially among seniors who may have mobility challenges or prefer the convenience of virtual interactions. Platforms such as BetterHelp and Talkspace offer access to licensed therapists who specialize in mental health issues faced by older adults. These services can provide tailored support for those dealing with the emotional burdens of diabetes, including fear of complications and lifestyle adjustments. By utilizing these resources, seniors can address their mental health concerns in a comfortable and accessible manner.

Finally, educational books and resources focusing on diabetes management often include sections on mental health. Publications from reputable organizations, such as the American Diabetes Association, can provide insights into managing the psychological aspects of diabetes. These materials can help seniors understand the interplay between diabetes and mental health, equipping them with tools to improve their overall quality of life. By leveraging these various resources, diabetic seniors can take proactive steps toward maintaining their mental well-being, ultimately enhancing their journey toward living well with diabetes.

Chapter 9: Creating a Diabetes Management Plan

Setting Realistic Goals

Setting realistic goals is a crucial step for diabetic seniors aiming to manage their health effectively. Goals should be specific, measurable, achievable, relevant, and time-bound (SMART). This approach ensures that the objectives you set are not only clear but also attainable within a certain timeframe. For instance, instead of aiming to "eat healthier," a more specific goal might be to "include at least two servings of vegetables in every meal." This clarity helps in tracking progress and making necessary adjustments.

When setting goals, it is essential to consider individual circumstances, including existing health conditions, lifestyle, and support systems. Each person's journey with diabetes is unique, and what may work for one individual may not be suitable for another. Therefore, it is advisable to involve healthcare professionals, such as doctors, dietitians, or diabetes educators, who can provide personalized advice and help tailor goals to fit personal health needs. Collaborating with healthcare providers can yield more effective and realistic objectives.

Another important aspect of goal setting is to focus on gradual changes rather than drastic shifts. Rapid changes in lifestyle can be overwhelming and may lead to frustration or burnout. For example, instead of drastically reducing carbohydrate intake overnight, consider setting a goal to reduce it by a small amount each week. This gradual approach allows for better adaptation and increases the likelihood of sustaining new habits over the long term. It also provides opportunities to celebrate small successes along the way, which can motivate continued progress.

In addition to dietary goals, it is vital to incorporate physical activity into your routines. Setting achievable fitness goals, such as walking for 10 minutes a day and gradually increasing that time, can improve overall health and well-being. Physical activity has numerous benefits for diabetic seniors, including better blood sugar control, enhanced mood, and increased energy levels. Engaging in regular exercise can also serve as a motivating factor when setting and achieving other health-related goals.

Finally, it is essential to regularly review and adjust your goals as needed. Life can be unpredictable, and various factors such as health changes, social circumstances, or personal preferences may influence your ability to stick to your initial plans. Periodic evaluations of your goals allow you to recognize achievements, identify challenges, and adapt your objectives accordingly. This flexibility promotes a more positive experience in managing diabetes, fostering a sense of control and empowerment over one's health. By setting realistic goals, diabetic seniors can take significant steps toward living well and maintaining a healthy lifestyle.

Working with Healthcare Teams

Working with healthcare teams is a crucial aspect of managing diabetes effectively, especially for seniors. As you navigate the complexities of your condition, it is important to understand that you are not alone. A healthcare team typically consists of various professionals, including your primary care physician, endocrinologist, dietitian, diabetes educator, and sometimes even a mental health counselor. Each member of this team plays a unique role in your care, and collaborating with them can significantly enhance your well-being.

Communication is key when working with healthcare teams. It is essential to be open and honest about your symptoms, lifestyle, and any challenges you face in managing your diabetes. This information enables your healthcare providers to tailor their advice and treatment plans to suit your individual needs. Regular check-ins with your team members allow for adjustments in your care plan based on your progress or any changes in your health status. Make it a habit to prepare questions or topics you want to discuss during your appointments to maximize the time spent with your healthcare providers.

Understanding the roles of each team member can also improve your experience with healthcare. Your primary care physician often serves as the coordinator of your care, managing your overall health and referring you to specialists as needed. The endocrinologist focuses on hormone-related issues, including insulin management. A registered dietitian can help you create a meal plan that aligns with your dietary needs, while a diabetes educator can provide you with the necessary skills to monitor your blood sugar levels effectively. Recognizing these roles allows you to engage more meaningfully with each professional, creating a more cohesive approach to your diabetes management.

Empowerment is another vital component of working with healthcare teams. As a senior, you bring valuable insights into your own health and experiences. It's important to advocate for yourself and express any concerns you may have about your treatment options. This empowerment fosters a collaborative spirit, where your preferences and values are taken into account when developing your care plan. Remember that you have the right to ask for clarification and seek second opinions if necessary, ensuring that you are comfortable and confident in the decisions being made regarding your health.

Finally, building a strong relationship with your healthcare team can lead to better health outcomes. Trust and rapport are essential, as they foster an environment where you feel comfortable discussing personal aspects of your life that may affect your diabetes management. Regular follow-ups and open lines of communication can help establish this relationship. You might also consider involving family members or caregivers in your healthcare discussions, as they can provide additional support and help you remember important information. Together, a

united healthcare team can empower you to live well with diabetes, making informed choices that enhance your quality of life.

Adapting to Changes Over Time

Adapting to changes over time is crucial for diabetic seniors as they navigate the complexities of managing their health. As individuals age, their bodies undergo various physiological changes that can impact diabetes management. These changes may include decreased insulin sensitivity, alterations in metabolism, and the presence of other chronic conditions. Understanding these factors can help seniors make informed decisions about their care, ensuring that they adapt their lifestyle and treatment plans to meet their evolving needs.

One significant change that many seniors experience is a shift in their physical activity levels. With age, mobility may decline due to joint issues, muscle weakness, or other health concerns. It is essential for diabetic seniors to find appropriate forms of exercise that suit their capabilities while still providing cardiovascular benefits and aiding blood sugar control. Activities such as walking, swimming, or gentle yoga can be excellent options. Engaging in regular physical activity not only helps manage diabetes but also supports overall health, improves mood, and enhances quality of life.

Dietary needs also evolve over time, necessitating careful attention to nutrition. As metabolism slows and appetite may fluctuate, it becomes important for seniors to focus on nutrient-dense foods that promote stable blood sugar levels. Incorporating plenty of vegetables, lean proteins, whole grains, and healthy fats can provide the necessary fuel without excessive calories. Additionally, seniors should be mindful of portion sizes and consider working with a registered dietitian to develop meal plans that cater to their individual health goals and preferences.

Medication management is another area where adaptation is vital. As health conditions change, seniors may find that their diabetes medications need to be adjusted or that new medications are introduced to address other health issues. Regular consultations with healthcare providers can help ensure that treatment plans remain effective and safe. It is important for seniors to maintain open communication with their doctors about any side effects or concerns they may have regarding their medications, as this will facilitate timely adjustments as needed.

Lastly, the social and emotional aspects of living with diabetes can change over time. Seniors may face challenges related to isolation, the loss of loved ones, or the stress of managing multiple health conditions. Building a strong support network can be invaluable, whether through family, friends, or community resources. Participating in diabetes education programs or support

groups can also provide encouragement and practical advice from others facing similar challenges. Adapting to these emotional shifts is essential for maintaining a positive outlook and a proactive approach to living well with diabetes.

Celebrating Achievements

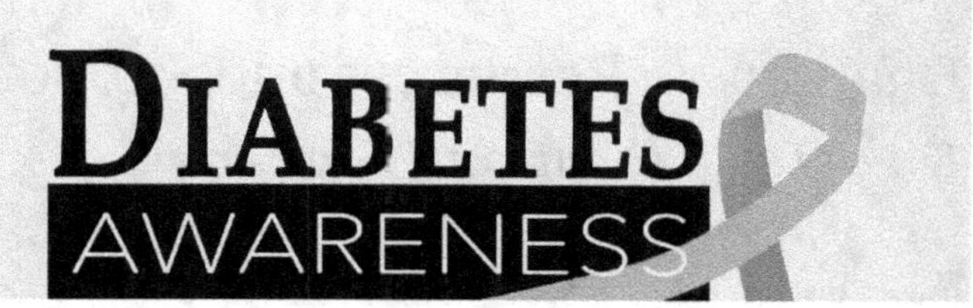

Celebrating achievements is an essential aspect of managing diabetes, particularly for seniors. Recognizing personal milestones can boost motivation, enhance self-esteem, and foster a positive outlook on life. Achievements can range from successfully maintaining blood sugar levels within target ranges, to adopting a healthier diet, or engaging in regular physical activity. Each of these accomplishments, no matter how small, contributes to better health outcomes and overall well-being.

One significant achievement for diabetic seniors is the ability to manage their diet effectively. Adopting a balanced diet that includes whole grains, lean proteins, healthy fats, and plenty of fruits and vegetables is a commendable feat. It involves planning meals, reading food labels, and understanding portion sizes. Celebrating this achievement can be done by sharing healthy recipes with friends and family, or even hosting a healthy cooking class. This not only reinforces the habit but also encourages social interaction, which is beneficial for mental health.

Another crucial area for celebration is physical activity. For many seniors, incorporating regular exercise into their routine can be challenging due to mobility issues or other health concerns. Yet, achieving consistent physical activity, whether through walking, swimming, or participating in senior fitness classes, deserves recognition. Seniors can celebrate this milestone by setting up a walking group with peers, tracking their exercise progress, or rewarding themselves with a new piece of workout gear. These activities not only enhance physical health but also provide a sense of community and support.

Monitoring blood sugar levels is a fundamental part of diabetes management, and achieving stable readings can be a significant accomplishment. For seniors, this often requires dedication to daily routines and adherence to medication regimens. Celebrating success in this area can involve sharing results with healthcare providers, who can provide positive reinforcement, or creating a visual chart at home to track progress. Additionally, establishing a regular check-in with a healthcare professional can help seniors feel more accountable and supported in their journey.

Lastly, emotional and mental well-being is a vital aspect of living well with diabetes. Seniors who take steps to manage stress, seek support, and engage in enjoyable activities are making significant strides. Celebrating these achievements could involve participating in community events, joining a support group, or engaging in hobbies that bring joy and fulfillment.

Acknowledging the importance of mental health not only reinforces the connection between mind and body but also encourages a holistic approach to living well with diabetes.

Chapter 10: Resources and Support
Diabetes Education Programs

Diabetes education programs play a crucial role in empowering seniors to manage their conditioneffectively.Theseprogramsaredesignedtoprovideessentialinformationabout diabetes, including its causes, symptoms, and potential complications. For seniors, understanding how diabetes affects their bodies can lead to better health outcomes. These programs often cover key topics such as blood sugar monitoring, the importance of diet and nutrition, physical activity, and medication management. By participating in these educational initiatives, seniors can gain the knowledge they need to make informed decisions about their health.

One of the primary benefits of diabetes education programs is the opportunity for seniors to learn about dietary management specific to their needs. Nutrition plays a vital role in managing blood glucose levels, and these programs often include guidance on meal planning, carbohydrate counting, and reading food labels. Seniors can benefit from learning how to prepare healthy meals that cater to their dietary restrictions while still being enjoyable. By understanding the relationship between food choices and blood sugar levels, seniors can take control of their condition and improve their overall health.

Physical activity is another critical aspect addressed in diabetes education programs. Many seniors face mobility challenges that may limit their ability to engage in regular exercise. However, these programs often provide tailored recommendations for safe and effective physical activities suitable for seniors. Participants can learn about the benefits of incorporating gentle exercises such as walking, swimming, or chair yoga into their daily routines. Engaging in regular physical activity can help seniors manage their weight, improve insulin sensitivity, and enhance their overall quality of life.

Medication management is also a significant component of diabetes education. Seniors often take multiple medications for various health conditions, which can complicate diabetes management. Education programs typically cover how to properly administer medications, understand their effects, and recognize potential side effects. Seniors are encouraged to maintain open communication with their healthcare providers to ensure that their diabetes medications are optimized for their specific health profiles. This knowledge can lead to better adherence to treatment plans and ultimately reduce the risk of complications.

Finally, diabetes education programs foster a supportive community where seniors can connect with others facing similar challenges. Sharing experiences and tips can be invaluable in navigating the complexities of living with diabetes. Many programs offer group sessions where seniors can discuss their concerns, celebrate successes, and motivate each other to stay on track with their health goals. Building a network of support not only enhances the educational experience but also helps seniors feel less isolated and more empowered in their journey to live well with diabetes.

Online Resources and Communities

The internet offers a wealth of resources specifically designed to support seniors living with diabetes. Websites dedicated to diabetes management provide valuable information on nutrition, exercise, and medication management. Organizations such as the American Diabetes Association and Diabetes UK offer comprehensive guides, research updates, and tips tailored for seniors. These resources often include articles, webinars, and downloadable materials that can help seniors stay informed about the latest advancements in diabetes care. Bookmarking these sites can create a personalized hub of information that seniors can easily access.

Social media platforms have also emerged as vital tools for connecting seniors with diabetes. Facebook groups, for example, allow individuals to share their experiences, challenges, and successes in managing their condition. These online communities foster a sense of belonging and support, offering a space where members can ask questions, share recipes, and provide encouragement. Engaging in these discussions can help seniors feel less isolated and empower them to take a more active role in their health management.

Online forums and discussion boards dedicated to diabetes offer another avenue for seniors to seek advice and share knowledge. Many of these platforms feature sections specifically for seniors, addressing unique challenges such as memory issues, mobility concerns, or co-existing health conditions. Participants can post questions and receive responses from peers who have faced similar situations, creating a rich tapestry of shared wisdom. This peer-to-peer support can be invaluable, especially for those who may not have immediate family members nearby to discuss their health concerns.

In addition to community support, there are numerous apps and tools designed to assist seniors in managing their diabetes. Many of these applications allow users to track their blood sugar levels, monitor their diet, and set medication reminders. Some apps even provide educational resources, including meal planning suggestions and exercise routines tailored to seniors. By utilizing these digital tools, seniors can take charge of their health in a more organized and informed manner, leading to better diabetes management outcomes.

Lastly, online health webinars and virtual workshops can be beneficial for seniors seeking to deepen their understanding of diabetes care. Many healthcare institutions and diabetes organizations host these educational sessions, covering topics such as nutrition, managing

complications, and lifestyle modifications. Participating in these events can equip seniors with the knowledge they need to make informed decisions about their health. By actively engaging with online resources and communities, seniors can enhance their quality of life while effectively managing their diabetes.

Local Support Groups

Local support groups play a vital role in the lives of diabetic seniors, offering a space for sharing experiences, challenges, and successes. These groups provide an opportunity for individuals to connect with others who understand the unique struggles associated with managing diabetes. They foster a sense of community, reducing feelings of isolation and loneliness that can often accompany chronic health conditions. By coming together, members can share practical tips on managing blood sugar levels, dietary choices, and medication adherence, all while building meaningful relationships.

Participation in local support groups can significantly enhance emotional well-being. Diabetes management can be overwhelming, and having a network of peers who are facing similar challenges can provide much-needed encouragement. Members can exchange stories, celebrate milestones, and offer support during difficult times. This emotional connection can lead to improved mental health, which is crucial for overall well-being. Engaging in discussions about personal experiences also helps individuals feel validated, reinforcing the idea that they are not alone in their journey.

In addition to emotional support, local groups often host educational sessions led by healthcare professionals. These sessions can cover various topics, including nutrition, exercise, medication management, and coping strategies. Access to reliable information helps seniors make informed decisions about their health. It also empowers them to take control of their diabetes management, leading to better health outcomes. Furthermore, these educational opportunities can help dispel common myths about diabetes, ensuring that seniors have a clear understanding of their condition.

Moreover, local support groups can serve as a resource for finding additional services and programs within the community. Members often share information about workshops, fitness classes, and health screenings specifically designed for seniors with diabetes. This interconnectedness can help individuals stay active and engaged in their health management. By tapping into community resources, seniors can create a more comprehensive approach to maintaining their health, leading to a more fulfilling lifestyle.

Finally, involvement in local support groups can inspire a sense of accountability. When individuals regularly meet with others who are committed to managing their diabetes, it can motivate them to adhere to their health plans. Sharing goals with the group, tracking progress, and celebrating achievements together can encourage consistent efforts toward better health. By fostering a supportive environment where members hold each other accountable, local

support groups empower diabetic seniors to make healthier choices and maintain a positive outlook on their journey with diabetes.

Helpful Apps and Tools

In today's digital age, numerous apps and tools are designed to help individuals manage their diabetes more effectively. For diabetic seniors, these resources can provide essential support in monitoring blood sugar levels, tracking food intake, and managing medication schedules. Many of these applications are user-friendly and specifically cater to the needs of older adults, making them invaluable for maintaining a healthy lifestyle.

One of the most beneficial types of apps for seniors with diabetes is blood sugar monitoring tools. These applications allow users to log their glucose levels easily and analyze trends over time. Some apps even connect with glucose meters, automatically syncing readings for a more seamless experience. By keeping track of their blood sugar levels, seniors can make more informed decisions about their diet and activity levels, ultimately leading to better overall health management.

Nutrition tracking apps are another essential resource for diabetic seniors. These tools help users monitor their carbohydrate intake, identify healthy food options, and plan balanced meals. Many nutrition apps include extensive food databases, allowing seniors to quickly search for specific meals or ingredients and understand their nutritional content. This feature is particularly helpful for seniors who may have limited mobility or cooking abilities, as it empowers them to make healthier choices without extensive meal preparation.

Medication management apps can significantly reduce the risk of missed doses or medication errors for seniors managing multiple prescriptions. These tools offer reminders for taking medications on time and can track refills as well. Some applications even allow caregivers to monitor medication adherence, ensuring that seniors stay on track with their treatment plans. This support can be crucial for maintaining proper diabetes management and preventing complications associated with the disease.

Finally, support and community apps provide a platform for diabetic seniors to connect with others facing similar challenges. These applications often include forums, chat features, and access to health professionals who can offer advice and encouragement. Building a support network is vital for emotional well-being, and these tools can foster connections that help seniors feel less isolated in their diabetes journey. In conclusion, with the right combination of eating healthy, monitoring your blood sugar, exercising, using apps and tools, and following your doctor's advice;you can take proactive steps toward living well and maintaining a healthier life.

Celebrating Achievements

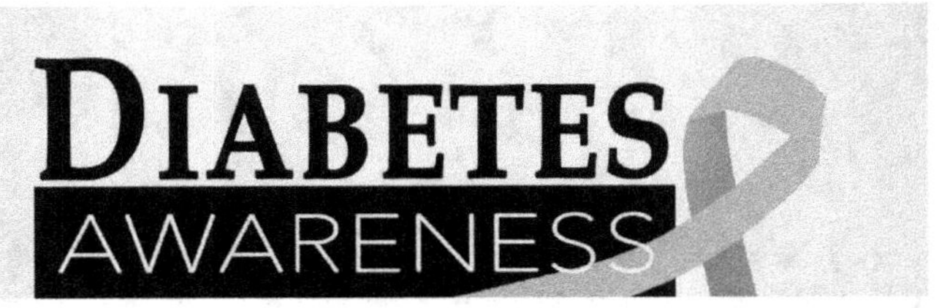

Celebrating achievements is an essential aspect of managing diabetes, particularly for seniors. Recognizing personal milestones can boost motivation, enhance self-esteem, and foster a positive outlook on life. Achievements can range from successfully maintaining blood sugar levels within target ranges, to adopting a healthier diet, or engaging in regular physical activity. Each of these accomplishments, no matter how small, contributes to better health outcomes and overall well-being.

One significant achievement for diabetic seniors is the ability to manage their diet effectively. Adopting a balanced diet that includes whole grains, lean proteins, healthy fats, and plenty of fruits and vegetables is a commendable feat. It involves planning meals, reading food labels, and understanding portion sizes. Celebrating this achievement can be done by sharing healthy recipes with friends and family, or even hosting a healthy cooking class. This not only reinforces the habit but also encourages social interaction, which is beneficial for mental health.

Another crucial area for celebration is physical activity. For many seniors, incorporating regular exercise into their routine can be challenging due to mobility issues or other health concerns. Yet, achieving consistent physical activity, whether through walking, swimming, or participating in senior fitness classes, deserves recognition. Seniors can celebrate this milestone by setting up a walking group with peers, tracking their exercise progress, or rewarding themselves with a new piece of workout gear. These activities not only enhance physical health but also provide a sense of community and support.

Monitoring blood sugar levels is a fundamental part of diabetes management, and achieving stable readings can be a significant accomplishment. For seniors, this often requires dedication to daily routines and adherence to medication regimens. Celebrating success in this area can involve sharing results with healthcare providers, who can provide positive reinforcement, or creating a visual chart at home to track progress. Additionally, establishing a regular check-in with a healthcare professional can help seniors feel more accountable and supported in their journey.

Lastly, emotional and mental well-being is a vital aspect of living well with diabetes. Seniors who take steps to manage stress, seek support, and engage in enjoyable activities are making significant strides. Celebrating these achievements could involve participating in community events, joining a support group, or engaging in hobbies that bring joy and fulfillment.

Acknowledging the importance of mental health not only reinforces the connection between mind and body but also encourages a holistic approach to living well with diabetes.

Chapter 10: Resources and Support
Diabetes Education Programs

Diabetes education programs play a crucial role in empowering seniors to manage their conditioneffectively.Theseprogramsaredesignedtoprovideessentialinformationabout diabetes, including its causes, symptoms, and potential complications. For seniors, understanding how diabetes affects their bodies can lead to better health outcomes. These programs often cover key topics such as blood sugar monitoring, the importance of diet and nutrition, physical activity, and medication management. By participating in these educational initiatives, seniors can gain the knowledge they need to make informed decisions about their health.

One of the primary benefits of diabetes education programs is the opportunity for seniors to learn about dietary management specific to their needs. Nutrition plays a vital role in managing blood glucose levels, and these programs often include guidance on meal planning, carbohydrate counting, and reading food labels. Seniors can benefit from learning how to prepare healthy meals that cater to their dietary restrictions while still being enjoyable. By understanding the relationship between food choices and blood sugar levels, seniors can take control of their condition and improve their overall health.

Physical activity is another critical aspect addressed in diabetes education programs. Many seniors face mobility challenges that may limit their ability to engage in regular exercise. However, these programs often provide tailored recommendations for safe and effective physical activities suitable for seniors. Participants can learn about the benefits of incorporating gentle exercises such as walking, swimming, or chair yoga into their daily routines. Engaging in regular physical activity can help seniors manage their weight, improve insulin sensitivity, and enhance their overall quality of life.

Medication management is also a significant component of diabetes education. Seniors often take multiple medications for various health conditions, which can complicate diabetes management. Education programs typically cover how to properly administer medications, understand their effects, and recognize potential side effects. Seniors are encouraged to maintain open communication with their healthcare providers to ensure that their diabetes medications are optimized for their specific health profiles. This knowledge can lead to better adherence to treatment plans and ultimately reduce the risk of complications.

Finally, diabetes education programs foster a supportive community where seniors can connect with others facing similar challenges. Sharing experiences and tips can be invaluable in navigating the complexities of living with diabetes. Many programs offer group sessions where seniors can discuss their concerns, celebrate successes, and motivate each other to stay on track with their health goals. Building a network of support not only enhances the educational experience but also helps seniors feel less isolated and more empowered in their journey to live well with diabetes.

Local Support Groups

Local support groups play a vital role in the lives of diabetic seniors, offering a space for sharing experiences, challenges, and successes. These groups provide an opportunity for individuals to connect with others who understand the unique struggles associated with managing diabetes. They foster a sense of community, reducing feelings of isolation and loneliness that can often accompany chronic health conditions. By coming together, members can share practical tips on managing blood sugar levels, dietary choices, and medication adherence, all while building meaningful relationships.

Participation in local support groups can significantly enhance emotional well-being. Diabetes management can be overwhelming, and having a network of peers who are facing similar challenges can provide much-needed encouragement. Members can exchange stories, celebrate milestones, and offer support during difficult times. This emotional connection can lead to improved mental health, which is crucial for overall well-being. Engaging in discussions about personal experiences also helps individuals feel validated, reinforcing the idea that they are not alone in their journey.

In addition to emotional support, local groups often host educational sessions led by healthcare professionals. These sessions can cover various topics, including nutrition, exercise, medication management, and coping strategies. Access to reliable information helps seniors make informed decisions about their health. It also empowers them to take control of their diabetes management, leading to better health outcomes. Furthermore, these educational opportunities can help dispel common myths about diabetes, ensuring that seniors have a clear understanding of their condition.

Moreover, local support groups can serve as a resource for finding additional services and programs within the community. Members often share information about workshops, fitness classes, and health screenings specifically designed for seniors with diabetes. This interconnectedness can help individuals stay active and engaged in their health management. By tapping into community resources, seniors can create a more comprehensive approach to maintaining their health, leading to a more fulfilling lifestyle.

Finally, involvement in local support groups can inspire a sense of accountability. When individuals regularly meet with others who are committed to managing their diabetes, it can motivate them to adhere to their health plans. Sharing goals with the group, tracking progress, and celebrating achievements together can encourage consistent efforts toward better health. By fostering a supportive environment where members hold each other accountable, local

Local Support Groups

Local support groups play a vital role in the lives of diabetic seniors, offering a space for sharing experiences, challenges, and successes. These groups provide an opportunity for individuals to connect with others who understand the unique struggles associated with managing diabetes. They foster a sense of community, reducing feelings of isolation and loneliness that can often accompany chronic health conditions. By coming together, members can share practical tips on managing blood sugar levels, dietary choices, and medication adherence, all while building meaningful relationships.

Participation in local support groups can significantly enhance emotional well-being. Diabetes management can be overwhelming, and having a network of peers who are facing similar challenges can provide much-needed encouragement. Members can exchange stories, celebrate milestones, and offer support during difficult times. This emotional connection can lead to improved mental health, which is crucial for overall well-being. Engaging in discussions about personal experiences also helps individuals feel validated, reinforcing the idea that they are not alone in their journey.

In addition to emotional support, local groups often host educational sessions led by healthcare professionals. These sessions can cover various topics, including nutrition, exercise, medication management, and coping strategies. Access to reliable information helps seniors make informed decisions about their health. It also empowers them to take control of their diabetes management, leading to better health outcomes. Furthermore, these educational opportunities can help dispel common myths about diabetes, ensuring that seniors have a clear understanding of their condition.

Moreover, local support groups can serve as a resource for finding additional services and programs within the community. Members often share information about workshops, fitness classes, and health screenings specifically designed for seniors with diabetes. This interconnectedness can help individuals stay active and engaged in their health management. By tapping into community resources, seniors can create a more comprehensive approach to maintaining their health, leading to a more fulfilling lifestyle.

Finally, involvement in local support groups can inspire a sense of accountability. When individuals regularly meet with others who are committed to managing their diabetes, it can motivate them to adhere to their health plans. Sharing goals with the group, tracking progress, and celebrating achievements together can encourage consistent efforts toward better health. By fostering a supportive environment where members hold each other accountable, local

support groups empower diabetic seniors to make healthier choices and maintain a positive outlook on their journey with diabetes.

Helpful Apps and Tools

In today's digital age, numerous apps and tools are designed to help individuals manage their diabetes more effectively. For diabetic seniors, these resources can provide essential support in monitoring blood sugar levels, tracking food intake, and managing medication schedules. Many of these applications are user-friendly and specifically cater to the needs of older adults, making them invaluable for maintaining a healthy lifestyle.

One of the most beneficial types of apps for seniors with diabetes is blood sugar monitoring tools. These applications allow users to log their glucose levels easily and analyze trends over time. Some apps even connect with glucose meters, automatically syncing readings for a more seamless experience. By keeping track of their blood sugar levels, seniors can make more informed decisions about their diet and activity levels, ultimately leading to better overall health management.

Nutrition tracking apps are another essential resource for diabetic seniors. These tools help users monitor their carbohydrate intake, identify healthy food options, and plan balanced meals. Many nutrition apps include extensive food databases, allowing seniors to quickly search for specific meals or ingredients and understand their nutritional content. This feature is particularly helpful for seniors who may have limited mobility or cooking abilities, as it empowers them to make healthier choices without extensive meal preparation.

Medication management apps can significantly reduce the risk of missed doses or medication errors for seniors managing multiple prescriptions. These tools offer reminders for taking medications on time and can track refills as well. Some applications even allow caregivers to monitor medication adherence, ensuring that seniors stay on track with their treatment plans. This support can be crucial for maintaining proper diabetes management and preventing complications associated with the disease.

Finally, support and community apps provide a platform for diabetic seniors to connect with others facing similar challenges. These applications often include forums, chat features, and access to health professionals who can offer advice and encouragement. Building a support network is vital for emotional well-being, and these tools can foster connections that help seniors feel less isolated in their diabetes journey. In conclusion, with the right combination of eating healthy, monitoring your blood sugar, exercising, using apps and tools, and following your doctor's advice;you can take proactive steps toward living well and maintaining a healthier life.

Conclusion

In conclusion, "Healthy Guide for Seniors with Diabetes" aims to empower seniors with the knowledge and tools necessary to maintain a fulfilling and healthy lifestyle while managing diabetes. By embracing balanced nutrition, regular physical activity, and mindful self-care, seniors can effectively control their blood sugar levels, reduce complications, and enhance overall well-being. This guide also underscores the importance of regular medical check-ups and fostering a supportive network of healthcare professionals, family, and friends. Remember, managing diabetes is a journey, and while challenges may arise, the strategies and insights provided in this book can serve as a reliable compass, guiding you towards a healthier, more vibrant life. Let this guide be your companion in celebrating the possibilities of well-managed diabetes and the joyful years ahead.

Here are some extra tools, to encourage you along the way.

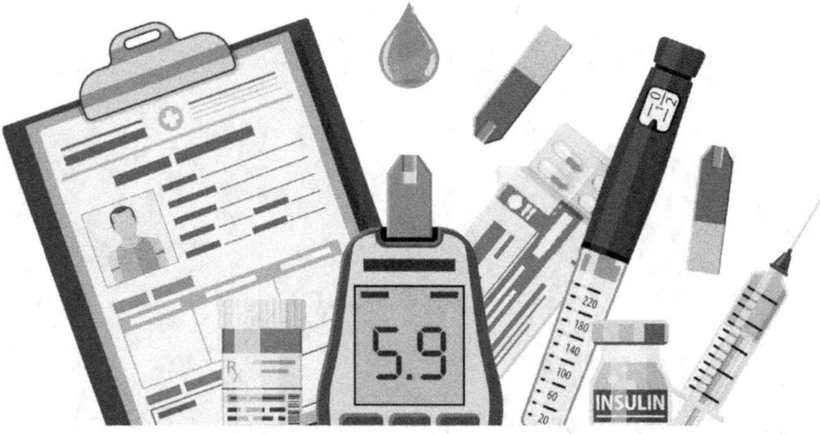

your Blood Sugar everyday.
Remember to log your numbers
for Doctor's visits.
Let's stay alert and monitor

THANK YOU!

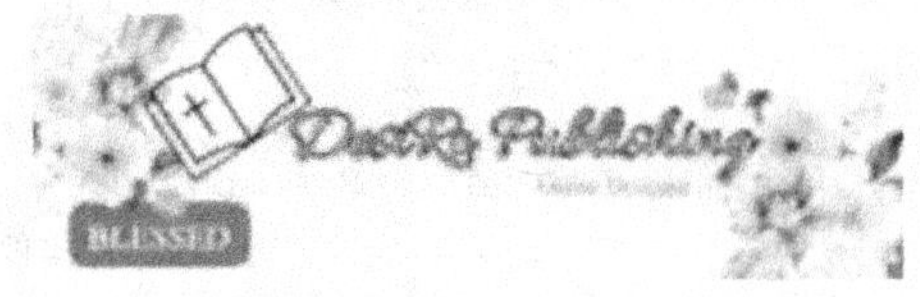

To My Readers

Thank you for buying my book I hope that this guide helps you to understand diabetes a little better,and helps you along the way.